Eternal Youth

The Ultimate Guide to Achieving Lifelong Health and Vitality

By
Dr. Brian Richter

Content

Introduction

Humans have always found the concept of endless youth to be fascinating. We have been looking for solutions to preserve our young energy and vitality since the time of the Fountain of Youth stories in antiquity. Aging is a natural process that cannot be totally prevented, but there are some lifestyle choices and activities that may help us retain our health and vigor for the rest of our lives.

Many scientific and medical developments have been sparked by the search for perpetual youth. Everything from the genetics of aging to the impact of diet and exercise on the aging process has been investigated by researchers. New treatments and therapies that can support us in preserving our health and vitality have been developed as a result of these investigations.

Nonetheless, despite these developments, the idea of everlasting youth is still unattainable. Changes occur at the molecular, cellular, and systemic levels as a result of aging, which is a complicated process. There is no one action that can entirely stop or reverse the aging process, even while some components of it can be slowed down or postponed.

This does not imply, however, that we should abandon our efforts to maintain our health and vigor throughout our lives. We may boost our general quality of life, our physical and mental health, and our risk of chronic illnesses by implementing healthy lifestyle behaviors. A balanced diet, regular exercise, sufficient sleep, stress management, maintaining social connections, and decent cleanliness are some of these behaviors.

One of the most crucial elements in preserving health and vigor for the rest of one's life is a well-balanced diet. The vital elements our bodies require to operate effectively may be obtained through a varied diet that includes fruits, vegetables, whole grains, lean meats, and healthy fats. Also, drinking lots of water to keep hydrated is crucial for sustaining general health.

For the purpose of preserving both physical and mental health, regular exercise is also crucial. Exercise promotes cardiovascular health, muscular growth and maintenance, stress and anxiety reduction, and better sleep. For optimum health, experts advise engaging in at least 150 minutes of moderate-intensity aerobic activity or 75 minutes of vigorous-intensity aerobic activity per week.

Another key element in preserving health and vigor for the rest of one's life is getting adequate sleep. Sleep is necessary for physical and mental rejuvenation. Obesity, diabetes, cardiovascular disease, and mental health problems are just a few of the health concerns that can develop as a result of obtaining poor sleep or not enough sleep.

Maintaining top health and wellness also requires effective stress management. Finding efficient techniques to manage stress is crucial since chronic stress can cause a number of health issues. Exercise, mindfulness exercises like yoga or meditation, time spent in nature, and pastimes or activities that make you happy and calm are some examples of this.

Maintaining relationships and social networks is crucial for overall welfare and mental health. Having supportive social networks can lower stress, elevate mood, and enhance general health. Spending time with friends and family, taking part in social events or clubs, or joining neighborhood or local organizations may all help you stay socially connected.

Lastly, using excellent hygiene can help to stop the transmission of germs and lower your chance of being sick. The risk of disease can be decreased by following good hygiene habits such as frequent hand washing, covering your mouth and nose when you cough or sneeze, and keeping surfaces clean.

Despite the fact that attaining eternal youth may be impossible, adopting good lifestyle habits can help you keep your health and vigor for the rest of your life. We may enhance our physical and mental health, lower our chance of developing chronic diseases, and improve our overall quality of life by eating a balanced diet, exercising frequently, getting adequate sleep, managing stress, maintaining social connections, and maintaining excellent cleanliness.

Chapter 1

A Balanced Diet

It is impossible to overestimate the significance of a balanced diet for maintaining good health and avoiding chronic illnesses. A balanced diet includes carbs, proteins, lipids, vitamins, minerals, and fiber, as well as all the other nutrients the body requires to operate at its best. A healthy diet should include fruits and vegetables as they include necessary vitamins, minerals, and fiber. To ensure a varied range of nutrients, it is advised to eat a variety of fruits and vegetables in various hues. For instance, berries like blueberries and strawberries are rich in antioxidants that help shield the body from cellular damage, while leafy greens like kale and spinach are high in iron and calcium.

Fiber, B vitamins, and other vital nutrients are found in whole grains like brown rice, quinoa, and whole wheat bread. These grains are more nutrient-dense than refined grains like white rice and white bread because they have not been stripped of their nutrient-rich outer layer. Consuming whole grains can lower your chance of developing chronic conditions like diabetes, heart disease, and some forms of cancer.

The body's tissues must be built and repaired, which calls for lean proteins like those found in fish, poultry, and beans. Omega-3 fatty acids, which are abundant in fish in particular, can aid in reducing inflammation and lowering the risk of heart disease.Furthermore a fantastic source of fiber, which may help control blood sugar levels and encourage feelings of fullness, are plant-based proteins like beans and lentils.

Good fats, including those in nuts, seeds, and avocados, are crucial for maintaining healthy skin, hair, and brain function. These fats are also necessary for the absorption of several vitamins, including vitamin D and A. Limiting saturated and trans fats, which may be found in meals like fried dishes and rcd meat and raise the risk of chronic illnesses like heart disease, is vital.

A balanced diet is essential, but so is being mindful of portion sizes and avoiding processed foods and added sugars. Certain meals can lead to weight gain and raise the chance of developing chronic illnesses like diabetes and heart disease. Water serves to regulate body temperature, carry nutrients throughout the body, and eliminate waste, making it crucial to drink lots of it throughout the day in order to maintain general health.

In general, a balanced diet is crucial for good aging. We may promote our physical and mental health and lower our risk of chronic illnesses by eating a range of nutrient-rich meals. Our general health and wellness may be significantly impacted by making minor dietary adjustments, such as increasing our intake of fruits and vegetables, switching to whole grains instead of refined grains, and selecting lean meats and healthy fats.

Yes, of course! Consuming a balanced diet is vital for both physical and mental health. A diet rich in fruits, vegetables, whole grains, and lean proteins, while being low in processed foods and added sugars, has been demonstrated in research to help lessen the symptoms of sadness and anxiety. A diet high in omega-3 fatty acids, which are present in fatty fish and nuts, has also been demonstrated to enhance mood and cognitive performance. A balanced diet can make us feel better about our gut health in addition to supplying us with necessary nutrients. Trillions of bacteria that make up our gut microbiome are essential for digestion, immunological response, and general health.Consuming a diet high in fiber and fermented foods, like kimchi and yogurt, might aid in the growth of beneficial bacteria in our guts, which can lessen inflammation and enhance immunological performance.

Focusing on diversity and moderation is essential for keeping a balanced diet. Consuming a variety of foods can assist us make sure we are consuming all the necessary nutrients. Also, it's critical to use moderation because eating excessively might result in weight gain and other health issues.

Following dietary recommendations like the Mediterranean diet or the USDA's MyPlate is one approach to make sure we are eating a balanced diet.These recommendations outline the kinds and serving sizes of meals we should consume to keep our health in check. To create a customized nutrition plan, it is crucial to remember that everyone has distinct nutritional needs and to speak with a healthcare professional or registered dietitian.

In conclusion, maintaining lifetime health and vigor requires consuming a balanced diet. The necessary elements required for optimum health may be obtained through a diet high in fruits, vegetables, whole grains, lean proteins, and healthy fats. This type of diet can also help avoid chronic illnesses, maintain a healthy weight, and increase energy levels. Furthermore, emphasizing diversity and moderation can support obtaining all of the vital nutrients we require while preserving a healthy balance.

There are always more specifics and nuanced topics that might be discussed, even if I've already addressed the key points of the significance of a balanced diet. For instance, dietary concerns and particular nutritional requirements may change based on variables including age, sex, degree of exercise, and underlying medical issues. A balanced diet may be made utilizing a number of various foods and cuisines. It is also crucial to keep in mind that cultural and personal preferences may affect dietary choices. The capacity to maintain a balanced diet may also be influenced by education and access to nutritious foods, and initiatives to enhance food systems and encourage healthy eating patterns can benefit public health. Ultimately, a balanced diet is one of many elements of a healthy lifestyle, even if its significance cannot be emphasized. Maintaining general health and wellness also requires regular physical exercise, stress reduction, and appropriate rest.

We can meaningfully enhance our health and quality of life by making simple adjustments to our food and lifestyle.

Chapter 2

Regular Exercise

For preserving and enhancing bone density and muscle mass, it's also advised to incorporate strength training workouts at least two days a week. In addition to enhancing balance and lowering the risk of falls, exercise is particularly beneficial for older persons. Finding fun and long-lasting workout options is crucial when deciding on the best sort of exercise. This might range from running, cycling, or swimming to team sports, yoga, and group fitness sessions. The secret is to select activities that complement your interests and way of life and to gradually build up their duration and intensity over time.

Regular exercise has several advantages, one of which is its effect on mental health. Exercise has been demonstrated to enhance mood, lessen signs of anxiety and sadness, and boost self-esteem. This is believed to be a result of both the social and psychological advantages of engaging in physical activity, as well as the production of endorphins, which are natural mood enhancers.

Exercise also helps to lower the chance of developing chronic illnesses including diabetes, heart disease, and some kinds of cancer. Exercise can enhance insulin sensitivity, lower blood pressure, and lower cholesterol levels in addition to reducing inflammation in the body. These advantages are especially crucial for people who are more likely to experience these illnesses, such as those who are overweight or obese or have a family history of heart disease.

Exercise should be undertaken carefully, and people should speak with a healthcare professional before beginning a new fitness regimen, especially if they have any underlying medical concerns. Also, it's critical to put safety first when exercising by using the proper gear, drinking plenty of water, and gradually building up your endurance over time. In conclusion, frequent exercise is crucial for maintaining health and vigor throughout one's lifetime. Exercise can enhance cardiovascular health, lower stress and anxiety, increase sleep quality, and aid to maintain and grow muscle mass. It is advised to incorporate strength training activities at least twice per week and to strive for at least 150 minutes of moderate-intensity aerobic activity or 75 minutes of vigorous-intensity aerobic exercise each week. We may enjoy the many physical and mental health advantages of exercise by selecting activities we love and can sustain, considering safety, and consulting with healthcare professionals.

I've spoken about the primary advantages and suggestions for exercise, but there are always more specifics and nuances that may be discussed. For instance, different health issues, such as osteoporosis or arthritis, may benefit from different forms of exercise. It is also possible to talk about the function of exercise in managing weight and how it affects metabolism and energy balance.

It's also crucial to understand that exercise and physical activity are two different things. While planned exercise regimens are crucial, adding more movement to your day, for example, by using the stairs instead of the lift or taking a stroll while you're at work can also have a positive impact on your health. Finally, it's crucial to understand that leading a healthy lifestyle includes more than just exercising. A balanced diet, effective stress management, and sufficient sleep are also essential for preserving overall health and wellness. We may experience a lifetime of energy and wellbeing by incorporating regular physical exercise into our everyday lives and adopting a holistic approach to health and wellness.

Chapter 3

Get Adequate Sleep

For the sake of both our physical and mental wellbeing, we must get adequate sleep. Our bodies consolidate memories, repair and renew tissues, and release hormones that control hunger and development when we sleep. Our bodies and minds cannot perform at their best without proper sleep. Adults should get 7-8 hours of sleep each night, however individual requirements may differ. How much sleep a person requires varies depending on a variety of factors, including age, lifestyle, and underlying medical issues. Prioritizing sleep is crucial, as are developing good sleep routines including waking up and going to bed at the same time every day, setting up a calm atmosphere for sleeping, and avoiding coffee and alcohol just before bed.

Lack of sleep or poor quality sleep can have a serious detrimental impact on our health. Daytime weariness and sleepiness are two of the most well-known effects of sleep loss. This can affect our focus, judgment, and quickness, which can be harmful while handling heavy machinery or while driving a car.

Chronic sleep deprivation or poor sleep quality have also been related to a number of health issues in addition to these acute impacts. Poor sleep is particularly closely linked to obesity and weight gain because it can interfere with the hormones that control hunger and metabolism. Persistent sleep deprivation has been linked to an increased risk of type 2 diabetes, cardiovascular disease, and several cancers.

Poor sleep has a big impact on mental health as well. Persistent sleep deprivation can intensify symptoms of anxiety and depression in people who already have them, and it has been related to an increased risk of developing these diseases. Moreover, lack of sleep can make stress, irritability, and mood swings worse.

There are a number of ways that can help you get better quality and longer-lasting sleep. They include utilizing relaxation techniques like meditation or deep breathing, practicing good sleep hygiene like minimizing screen time before bed, establishing a peaceful sleeping environment, and getting treated for underlying sleep disorders like sleep apnea. Moreover, it should be noted that getting adequate sleep is crucial to preserving general health and wellbeing. To increase the quality of their sleep, adults should emphasize having 7-8 hours of sleep each night. It is crucial to take sleep seriously and seek assistance if necessary because chronic sleep deprivation or poor sleep quality can have substantial negative impacts on physical and mental health. We may enhance our health and wellness for years to come by making sleep a priority as an essential part of a healthy lifestyle.

There are a few more things that may be mentioned to underline how crucial obtaining enough sleep is. For instance, sleep deprivation or inadequate sleep can affect our immune system. Lack of sleep increases a person's susceptibility to diseases, such as the common cold and flu, according to studies. The body's capacity to heal from ailments and wounds can also be hampered by sleep deprivation.

In addition, sleep is essential for the creation of memories and for learning. Students and those in occupations that demand a lot of learning or mental processing need adequate sleep, especially because sleep is when the brain consolidates knowledge and memories from the previous day. The importance of sleep quality in addition to quantity should be emphasized. Even if a person is obtaining the recommended amount of sleep each night, poor-quality sleep can still have a negative impact on their health. This is why it's crucial to develop good sleeping habits and to get help if sleep issues persist. Overall, having adequate good sleep is crucial for preserving one's physical and mental well-being, boosting one's immune system, and improving learning and memory. We can benefit from deep, restorative sleep and enjoy better general health and wellness by prioritizing sleep as a part of a healthy lifestyle.

Chapter 4

Stress Management

Another good strategy to reduce stress is to keep up social contacts. We can feel supported and less lonely or alone, which are major drivers of stress, by spending time with friends and family. In fact, research indicates that those with strong social ties fare better than those who are socially isolated in terms of their mental and physical health.

Participating in local activities or organizations that match our interests is one method to maintain social connections. This could entail participating in community service, joining a sports team or club, or going to social events like parties or concerts. We may maintain relationships with friends and loved ones by using social media and other digital communication tools, especially when face-to-face encounters aren't always possible.

Setting limits and developing the ability to refuse requests when necessary are crucial aspects of social connection. Overcommitting oneself can result in feelings of overload and stress, so it's critical to put our needs first and scale back on our commitments as needed.

Self-care routines, in addition to social interaction, can aid with stress management. Included in this are practices like taking a warm bath, reading a book, or deep breathing exercises that encourage calmness and mindfulness. In order to control stress and advance general wellbeing, it is crucial to give self-care activities top priority in our daily routine.

And lastly, getting advice from a mental health expert might be beneficial in managing stress. A therapist or counselor can offer coping mechanisms and support in addressing any underlying mental health issues.

Ultimately, stress control is crucial for preserving the best possible health and wellness. We may efficiently manage stress and live a better, happier life by putting social interaction, self-care, and professional help when necessary first. The core causes of stress in our life must be found and addressed in addition to the aforementioned measures. Making adjustments to our daily schedules, work-life balance, or interpersonal connections may be necessary. For instance, it can be important to reevaluate job duties or establish limits with coworkers if work-related stress is a substantial cause of stress.

Positive thinking and appreciation exercises can also aid with stress management. Focusing on the positive aspects of our lives, such as our connections, successes, and inner resources, might help us change our perspective and feel less stressed and anxious.

It's crucial to keep in mind that stress management is a continuous process and may necessitate a variety of tactics. Stress may happen to everybody from time to time, and when it does, seeking help is a show of strength, not weakness. We may live a happier, more satisfying life by putting our physical, mental, and emotional well-being first and using efficient stress management techniques.

Chapter 5

Be Connected Socially

A great method to reduce stress and enhance general mental health and wellness is to take part in hobbies or relaxing activities. Hobbies are pursuits carried out for enjoyment and self-gratification as opposed to for a job or other duty. They provide us the chance to partake in enjoyable activities, exhibit our creativity, and feel a feeling of success. Interests might include anything from gardening and reading to art, music, and hiking.

Engaging in leisure pursuits or activities that make you happy and relaxed can help to lower stress and enhance your feeling of wellness. Hobbies provide us the chance to focus on something other than our everyday obligations, relaxing our brains and fostering a sense of serenity.Drawing or painting are examples of artistic pursuits that may be peaceful and encourage awareness.

Hobbies and leisure time pursuits may reduce stress while also giving a sense of achievement and direction. We may elevate our mood, build self-esteem, and raise general life satisfaction by doing things we like. Joining a club or group activity can also provide you the chance to make new friends and strengthen existing ones, which can further enhance your mental health and wellness.

Prioritizing hobbies and leisure pursuits as a regular component of our routine is crucial. This may be setting out time each week for a cherished activity or experimenting with new things.As opposed to feeling forced to engage in activities that do not provide joy or relaxation, it is crucial to pick fun and gratifying hobbies.

Maintaining social connections is crucial for overall welfare and mental health. Social relationships offer emotional support, a sense of community, and can lessen feelings of isolation and loneliness. Spending time with friends and family, taking part in clubs or social activities, or joining neighborhood or civic organizations are all examples of how to do this.

Participation in organizations or group activities may be very helpful for fostering social connections and minimizing feelings of isolation. This might entail signing up for a neighborhood sports team, attending a reading club, or giving back to the neighborhood by volunteering.Meeting new individuals with comparable interests and beliefs through these activities fosters a feeling of community and social connectedness.

In conclusion, maintaining social connections and taking part in enjoyable, stress-relieving activities are crucial for enhancing overall mental health and wellness. We may lower stress, elevate mood, and foster a sense of purpose and satisfaction in our lives by making leisure time and social interactions a priority in our daily routine. A sense of purpose and fulfillment in life may be gained through hobbies and activities that are enjoyable and relaxing in addition to the advantages already discussed. Having a hobby or passion may make you feel accomplished and can also help you learn new things. It can also give a chance to meet others who have similar interests, whether through groups or online forums.

It is crucial to remember that everyone has different interests and pastimes that they find enjoyable and relaxing. Some people may find relaxation in reading, while others may find it in gardening or painting. To determine what interests and activities are ideal for you, it is vital to experiment.Including interests and pastimes in your everyday routine can also aid in stress management and relaxation. It might be as easy as setting up a short period of time each day to partake in an enjoyable activity, like listening to music or going for a stroll in the outdoors.

In general, taking part in enjoyable, stress-relieving activities may significantly improve both mental and physical health. It may lift one's spirits, lessen stress, give one a feeling of direction and fulfillment, and enhance general welfare.

Another thing to think about is that having enjoyable, stress-relieving hobbies or pastimes might help you achieve a better work-life balance. Many people get completely engrossed by their jobs or other obligations, which causes stress and burnout. They may maintain a feeling of balance in their life and avoid burnout by embracing hobbies and extracurricular activities.

In addition, engaging in hobbies and activities may help with self-care, which is crucial for preserving general health and wellness. Self-care is looking after one's physical, mental, and emotional well-being. It also includes participating in enjoyable and relaxing activities. In conclusion, finding joy and relaxation in pastimes or interests is important for preserving general health and wellness. It offers a sense of fulfilment and purpose, lowers stress, encourages relaxation, and may result in a better work-life balance. To get the most out of your daily routine and to reap the most health advantages, it's crucial to experiment with a variety of hobbies and interests.

Chapter 6

Good Practice of Hygiene

Maintaining excellent cleanliness is essential for preserving health and halting the spread of diseases. Regular hand washing is one easy way to drastically lower your risk of contracting and spreading germs. When there is a pandemic, as COVID-19, or during flu season, this is very crucial. It is advised to wash your hands for at least 20 seconds with soap and water, especially after using the lavatory or touching a common surface. You should also wash your hands before and after eating.

Covering your mouth and nose when sneezing or coughing is an additional crucial component of excellent hygiene. By doing this, the transmission of pathogens via breathing droplets can be stopped. While coughing or sneezing, it is advised to use a tissue and dispose of it correctly. In the absence of a tissue, sneeze or cough into your elbow or upper sleeve as opposed to your hands.

Surface cleanliness is crucial for preserving good hygiene. Because germs may remain alive on surfaces for several hours, there is a higher chance that diseases will spread. Germs may be stopped from spreading by routinely disinfecting surfaces like doorknobs, counters, and shared items like phones or keyboards.

Taking care of one's personal hygiene is part of maintaining healthy hygiene. This include routines like taking frequent showers or baths, cleaning your teeth twice a day, and dressing in clean clothes. These procedures can aid in preventing the growth of germs and the development of smells. Also, maintaining proper cleanliness might benefit mental wellness. A higher overall sense of wellbeing can result from feeling clean and refreshed, which can also increase self-worth and confidence.

In general, keeping excellent cleanliness is crucial for preserving health and stopping the spread of diseases. The danger of contracting and transmitting germs can be dramatically decreased by taking simple precautions including washing hands, covering mouth and nose when coughing or sneezing, and maintaining clean surfaces. Maintaining good personal cleanliness might benefit mental health as well. For the best possible health outcomes, it's crucial to develop healthy hygiene habits and incorporate them into everyday activities. In order to protect their health and stop the spread of disease, people can adopt additional basic hygiene habits into their everyday routine. For instance, maintaining personal hygiene may be aided by routinely taking showers or baths, cleaning teeth twice day, and washing one's hair.

Also, it's critical to maintain proper cleanliness when handling and preparing food. To avoid the formation of bacteria, this entails completely cleaning hands before handling food, thoroughly cooking it, and keeping it at the appropriate temperature. Also, maintaining proper hygiene in public areas might lessen the transmission of disease. Carrying hand sanitizer or disinfectant wipes to wash down surfaces before contacting them, covering the mouth and nose while coughing or sneezing, and avoiding direct contact with ill people are some ways to do this.

In general, maintaining proper cleanliness is crucial to preserving health and halting the spread of disease. We may shield ourselves and others around us from hazardous germs and bacteria by implementing these easy behaviours into our daily routine.

Conclusion

It is a well-known reality that as we get older, our bodies change in a number of ways that may affect our health and happiness. While it is difficult to stop the natural ageing process, adopting good lifestyle habits can help you keep your health and energy for the rest of your life.

Nutritional Balance:

Eating a balanced, wholesome diet is among the most crucial things you can do for your health. Consuming a range of meals that provide your body the nutrients it needs to function correctly entails doing just that. Lean proteins, whole grains, a variety of fruits and vegetables, as well as heart-healthy fats, should all be present in a balanced diet. Limiting your consumption of processed foods, sugary beverages, and saturated fats is also crucial because they can all have a negative impact on your health.

Exercise Frequently:

Exercise is yet another essential element of preserving health and vigour for the rest of one's life. You may strengthen your muscles, strengthen your immune system, and enhance your cardiovascular health by engaging in regular physical activity. Also, it can assist you in maintaining a healthy weight and lower your chance of contracting chronic illnesses including diabetes, heart disease, and some types of cancer. Plan to engage in moderate activity for at least 30 minutes each day, such as brisk walking, cycling, or swimming.

Making Time for Sleep:

For sustaining excellent health and wellness, sleep is crucial. It enables your body to recuperate and heal itself, as well as helping to elevate your mood and sharpen your mind. To help your body get into a rhythm, try to establish a regular sleep schedule and aim for seven to nine hours of sleep each night.

Controlling Stress:

It's critical to learn appropriate coping mechanisms for stress because it may have a detrimental influence on your health. This might be engaging in mindfulness, meditation, yoga, or just finding relaxing things you love. Also, it's crucial to emphasise self-care activities that make you feel grounded and focused and to maintain a healthy work-life balance.

Maintaining Social Contact:

It's critical to maintain social connections since social isolation can be harmful to your health. Spending time with friends and family, participating in clubs or social organisations, and doing community service are a few examples of how to do this. Maintaining social connections may boost your mood, lower your risk of melancholy and anxiety, and foster a feeling of meaning and community.

Making Use of Excellent Hygiene:

For the transmission of disease and sickness to be stopped, proper hygiene habits are crucial. This entails often washing your hands, covering your mouth and nose when you sneeze or cough, and keeping your distance from other people when you're ill. To help stop the spread of infectious illnesses, it's necessary to be vaccinated, follow suggested health precautions, and get immunised.

Despite the fact that attaining eternal youth may be impossible, adopting good lifestyle habits can help you keep your health and vigour for the rest of your life. You may attain and preserve optimal health and wellbeing throughout your life by eating a balanced diet, exercising frequently, getting adequate sleep, managing stress, remaining socially engaged, and practising excellent hygiene. Never forget that it is never too late to begin making changes for a better and happy version of yourself.